I0696809

A Guide
to Childhood
Rheumatoid
Arthritis

A Guide to Childhood Rheumatoid Arthritis

Diagnosis, Treatment, and Support

Victor Asher

A Guide to Childhood Rheumatoid Arthritis

Diagnosis, Treatment, and Support

Victor Asher

Copyright © 2023 Victor Asher
All rights reserved
ISBN-13: 9798863261003

Other Book(s) by Victor Asher

The Role of Nutrition in Osteomyelitis Healing and Prevention

Dedication

This book is dedicated to God for His grace and wisdom, to my family, to my beautiful readers who will find this book relevant to them, and to everyone who has loved, supported, and encouraged me along the way. I would not be in the position I am in today without your unshakable faith in me. I dedicate this book to all my readers' especially those children with juvenile arthritis and I wish you all God's healing.

Table of Contents

Acknowledgement

I want to sincerely thank God for providing the means and insight that guided me during the writing of this book. I cannot forget my family members, whose encouragement and support have given me bravery and motivation throughout the process.

Thank you to my editor and publisher for their crucial advice and help in bringing this project to its successful conclusion. I would like to express my gratitude to everyone who so kindly contributed their time and knowledge to this project and added their wisdom. I want to express my gratitude to my friends as well, I appreciate all of your steadfast love and support throughout the journey.

I like to thank yummymummyclub.ca for the wonderful image, I really appreciate.

Finally, I extend my thanks to each and every one of you for purchasing and reading my work. I am thankful it met your needs and added to your knowledge. I sincerely value each and every one of you and think you're all fantastic.

Introduction

In the realm of pediatric healthcare, where stories of courage often outshine tales of adversity, there exists a journey both challenging and profoundly hopeful. It's a path traversed by children and families grappling with Juvenile Idiopathic Arthritis (JIA), a condition that casts shadows of uncertainty but is also illuminated by the light of understanding, effective treatments, and unwavering support.

Imagine a child's world suddenly touched by a condition that can bring joint pain, inflammation, and uncertainty. But also imagine that same child's world brightened by the promise of understanding, effective treatments, and unwavering support. Our journey through these pages begins with a quest to understand JIA: an intricate tapestry woven from history, shaped by prevalence, and enriched by the profound impact it leaves in its wake. To guide our exploration, let's first glimpse into the past.

Juvenile Idiopathic Arthritis, known affectionately as JIA, has its roots deep in the annals of medical history. While it wasn't officially christened until more recent times, the condition's existence has been acknowledged for well over a century. It was the pioneering pediatrician Frederick Still who, in 1896, first described this enigmatic ailment. However, it wasn't until 1946 that a specialized center for the study of Juvenile Rheumatism emerged, nestled in the heart of Berkshire, United Kingdom. This pivotal moment marked the beginning of a concerted effort to unravel the mysteries of JIA, a condition destined to leave an indelible mark on the lives of countless children and their families.

The prevalence of JIA, while relatively rare, is not to be underestimated. It affects approximately 1 in every 1,000 children under the age of 16. These numbers underscore the importance of comprehensive guidance and support, which is exactly what this book aims to provide.

As we venture further into the heart of JIA, we'll also explore a crucial pillar in its management: exercise. Far from being a mere footnote, exercise becomes a beacon of hope, offering strength and vitality. We'll delve into the significance of tailored exercise routines and techniques that empower young warriors to not only manage their condition but to thrive, body and spirit intertwined.

As we embark on this journey together, our mission is clear: to empower children with JIA and their families to face this condition with courage, knowledge, and the unwavering belief that a brighter tomorrow is not a distant dream but a reality within reach. This guide is not just a resource; it's a testament to the resilience of the human spirit when faced with adversity. Together, we'll navigate the path to understanding, treatment, and, ultimately, a life filled with hope, resilience, and boundless possibilities.

Welcome to "A Guide to Childhood Rheumatoid Arthritis: Diagnosis, Treatment, and Support," where knowledge and compassion unite to illuminate the path ahead.

Let's get started.

Chapter 1

Childhood Rheumatoid Arthritis

Childhood rheumatoid arthritis sometimes referred to as "pediatric rheumatic disease" or "juvenile rheumatoid arthritis" or "Juvenile arthritis" or "Still's disease" and currently "juvenile idiopathic arthritis", isn't a single, distinct illness. Instead, it serves as an overarching label for various inflammatory and rheumatic conditions that emerge in children below the age of 16.

These health issues collectively impact children and teenagers across the globe in a large percentage. It impacts around 1 in every 1,000 children and typically occurs in those under the age of 16. Importantly, JIA is generally not passed down through family inheritance. This condition is chronic in nature and can persist for several months or even years. However, the encouraging news is that approximately 75% of children with JRA eventually outgrow it.

Juvenile idiopathic arthritis (JIA) was first described by the dedicated pediatrician Frederick Still in 1896 at Great Ormond Street Hospital. However, it wasn't until 1946 that a dedicated center for researching juvenile rheumatism was established at the Canadian Red Cross Memorial Hospital in Taplow, Berkshire.

Since 1995, the preferred terms for childhood rheumatic arthritis have shifted from juvenile rheumatoid arthritis (JRA) and juvenile chronic arthritis (JCA) to juvenile idiopathic arthritis (JIA).

What then is this condition?

It is a condition in children marked by ongoing inflammation, leading to joint swelling, discomfort, and stiffness.

Many forms of JA fall under the categories of autoimmune or autoinflammatory conditions. In simpler terms, this means that the body's immune system, originally designed to defend against external threats like viruses and bacteria, becomes confused. It starts releasing inflammatory substances that mistakenly target and harm healthy cells and tissues. For most children with JA, this leads to symptoms like joint inflammation, swelling, pain, and tenderness.

However, there are certain JA types where joint symptoms are minimal or absent, and the condition may primarily impact the skin or internal organs."

Cause of Juvenile Idiopathic Arthritis (JIA)

Although the cause of JIA is not well known. However, they suspect that a combination of genetic factors and environmental influences plays a complex role in this process. This condition arises when the immune system triggers inflammation in the joint lining. Researchers have not yet pinpointed why the immune system targets healthy tissues in children with JIA.

In JIA, the body's immune system, which usually works to defend against infections and facilitate healing, erroneously targets some of its own healthy cells and tissues. This leads to inflammation, characterized by pain, swelling, warmth, and stiffness. The inflammation from JIA can potentially harm the joints, eyes, or other affected organs.

Inflammation is a process in which the immune system deploys signaling molecules and white blood cells to an area of injury or disease to combat invading microbes and aid in tissue repair. Typically, once healing is accomplished, the body halts the inflammatory response to safeguard its own cells and tissues from harm. However, individuals with juvenile idiopathic arthritis (JIA) experience prolonged inflammation, especially during joint movement. The precise reasons behind this excessive inflammatory response remain unclear.

Researchers have identified the changes in various genes that could influence the susceptibility of one to juvenile idiopathic arthritis. Some of these genes are part of the human leukocyte antigen (HLA) complex, which is responsible for producing a group of related proteins. This complex plays a crucial role in helping the immune system distinguish between the body's own proteins and those produced by external bodies, basically microorganisms like viruses and bacteria.

Each HLA gene has numerous different variations, enabling each individual's immune system to respond to a wide array of foreign bodies (proteins). Certain variations in several HLA genes appear to impact the risk of developing juvenile idiopathic arthritis and the specific subtype of the condition a person might develop.

In addition to changes in HLA genes, various other genes with natural variations have been linked to juvenile idiopathic arthritis, many of which are believed to be involved in immune system function. Moreover, there are likely to be other genetic factors that are yet unidentified, as well as environmental influences, such as infections and other factors affecting immune health, that collectively contribute to a person's likelihood of developing this intricate disorder.

Even though the exact cause of the immune system's excessive response in JIA remains uncertain, scientists have identified certain molecules that contribute to inflammation in certain forms of the disease. It's been discovered that three molecules play a role in generating joint inflammation in many children with JIA.
The molecules are:

- TNF-α (Tumour necrosis factor alpha)

It is a potent paracrine and endocrine mediator of inflammatory and immune functions.

- IL-6 (Interleukin 6)

Interleukin 6 (IL-6) is a type of interleukin that functions as both a pro-inflammatory cytokine and an anti-inflammatory myokine.

- IL-1 (Interleukin-1)

Interleukin-1 is a cytokine known for its strong inflammatory and immune-enhancing properties, primarily produced by macrophages as part of the body's defense responses. IL-1 is a proinflammatory cytokine that holds significance in promoting inflammation and contributing to the damage associated with rheumatoid arthritis (RA).

This discovery has paved the way for new treatments that specifically target these molecules.

Chapter 2

Types

There are several types of JIA, each characterized by its unique features. However, they typically share common symptoms such as joint pain, swelling, warmth, and stiffness that persist for a minimum of six weeks.

In 2001, the International League of Associations for Rheumatology (ILAR) convened a consensus conference to establish seven distinct categories for juvenile idiopathic arthritis (JIA).

They include:
1. Enthesitis-related arthritis
2. Psoriatic arthritis
3. Systemic arthritis
4. Undifferentiated arthritis
5. Rheumatoid factor (RF) positive polyarthritis
6. RF negative polyarthritis
7. Oligoarthritis

Let's look at them briefly:

1. Enthesitis-related Juvenile Idiopathic Arthritis

This variety of JIA involves arthritis and enthesitis. Enthesitis occurs when inflammation arises where a ligament or tendon connects to a bone. It primarily impacts the joints and attachment points of the lower limbs and can eventually extend to involve the sacroiliac joints and spine, progressing towards juvenile ankylosing spondylitis. The most common sites for enthesitis are the knees, heels, and the undersides of the feet.

Arthritis typically affects the hips, knees, ankles, and feet, but it can also lead to inflammation in the sacroiliac joints (located at the base of the back) and spinal joints. Some children may experience sudden episodes of acute anterior uveitis, which is inflammation at the front of the eye. Unlike most other forms of JIA, enthesitis-related JIA is more prevalent in boys.

Enthesitis-related juvenile idiopathic arthritis is also known as juvenile spondyloarthropathy.

2. Psoriatic Juvenile Idiopathic Arthritis

Psoriatic arthritis is a subtype of juvenile idiopathic arthritis (JIA) characterized by persistent joint inflammation and swelling. Additionally, there is an elevated risk of experiencing symptom-free eye inflammation.

Typically, the skin condition manifests initially, but in some cases, painful and stiff joints may be the initial indication, with the skin disorder emerging years later. Pitted fingernails and dactylitis, which involves swollen fingers or toes, are also indicative signs of the condition.

Psoriatic arthritis is a type of arthritis that occurs in certain individuals who have psoriasis, a chronic skin and nail condition known for causing red, scaly rashes and thick, pitted fingernails.

Approximately one-third of children with psoriasis will develop psoriatic arthritis.

Psoriatic arthritis represents roughly 6 percent of all instances of juvenile arthritis.

3. Systemic Juvenile Idiopathic Arthritis

"Systemic" indicates that the ailment can impact the entire body rather than targeting a specific organ such as the liver, lungs, and heart or joint. Systemic JIA typically commences with recurring fever and rash, lasting for a minimum of two weeks.

Systemic juvenile idiopathic arthritis (SJIA), also known as Still's disease, can manifest at any point during childhood, but it typically begins around the age of two. This condition affects both boys and girls equally. In numerous instances, joint inflammation follows, although it may occur much later after the fever subsides, or it might not occur at all if treatment is initiated promptly.

In more severe cases, inflammation can emerge in and around organs like the spleen, lymph nodes, liver, and the linings of the heart and lungs. Systemic JIA affects both boys and girls equally. SJIA is generally more severe and presents greater diagnostic and treatment challenges compared to other forms of juvenile idiopathic arthritis. For many patients, it's a lifelong condition that can persist into adulthood.

4. Undifferentiated Arthritis

Undifferentiated arthritis is a category that encompasses children with symptoms that don't align with any of the other specific types of juvenile idiopathic arthritis or those that may correspond to multiple types simultaneously. Undifferentiated arthritis" (UA) is just another way of saying early inflammatory arthritis. This means the illness hasn't fully taken shape yet, so it can't be specifically identified as a particular type of arthritis.

The term "undifferentiated arthritis" (UA) is employed to refer to individuals with early inflammatory arthritis, typically lasting between six weeks and a year, where the exact diagnosis or differentiation from other well-defined disorders is not yet clear. However, a diagnosis can often be established within three months, and only rarely does it take up to a year to become evident. Many of these patients will eventually receive a diagnosis of rheumatoid arthritis (RA) as their symptoms and findings further evolve.

According to a study by Schiff, published in the *American Journal of Managed Care* in 2010, roughly 40% to 50% of individuals with undifferentiated arthritis experience natural remission, where their symptoms resolve without treatment. Around 30% of those with this diagnosis eventually develop rheumatoid arthritis (RA), while the remaining 20% to 30% go on to develop various other forms of inflammatory arthritis.

5. Polyarticular Juvenile Idiopathic Arthritis (Rheumatoid Factor Positive).

Rheumatoid factor-positive polyarticular juvenile idiopathic arthritis, also known as polyarthritis with positive rheumatoid factor (when a blood test is conducted), is arthritis that leads to inflammation in five or more joints within the initial six months of the illness.

A child with this type has arthritis in five or more joints during the first 6 months of the disease. Tests for rheumatoid factor, a marker for autoimmune disease, are positive. It tends to occur in preteen and teenage girls, and it appears to be essentially the same as adult rheumatoid arthritis.

This form of arthritis closely resembles the rheumatoid arthritis observed in adults.

6. Polyarticular juvenile idiopathic arthritis (Rheumatoid Factor Negative).

This is the second most common type, involving inflammation in five or more joints within the first six months. Rheumatoid factor tests show negative. The rheumatoid factor blood test is used to check for autoimmune diseases, particularly rheumatoid arthritis, which is an adult form of arthritis. Some of these children may also develop chronic uveitis.

7. Oligoarticular juvenile idiopathic arthritis

Oligoarticular juvenile idiopathic arthritis, also known as oligoarthritis, is characterized by the presence of arthritis in four or fewer joints during the initial six months of the illness. It's divided into two subtypes based on the disease's progression.

If the arthritis remains in four or fewer joints after six months, it's classified as persistent oligoarthritis. If more than four joints are affected after six months, it's classified as extended oligoarthritis. Individuals with oligoarthritis have a higher risk of developing inflammation of the eye, known as uveitis.

The joints most commonly affected are the knees or ankles in this form of JIA. Children with this condition are also at risk of developing a long-lasting form of eye inflammation known as chronic uveitis. It's worth noting that about half of children with JIA have this type.

Chapter 3

Symptoms of JIA

JIA is a condition that affects children and adolescents, and it can have various symptoms. One of the most common signs is joint pain, which can be persistent and might come with swelling, warmth, and stiffness in the affected joints.

It's essential to pay attention to the typical signs and symptoms of childhood rheumatoid arthritis. These are like warning signs that something might be wrong and require immediate attention. They can make it tough for children or teenagers to move and carry out their daily tasks easily. Early detection and proper medical care are crucial to effectively manage the condition and its impact on their lives.

The symptoms include:

1. Joint Pain: Children with JIA often experience joint pain. It can range from mild discomfort to severe pain, and it usually affects multiple joints. The pain can be worse in the morning or after periods of inactivity.

2. Joint Swelling: Swelling in the joints is a typical sign of JIA. The affected joints may appear larger or feel warm to the touch due to inflammation.

3. Joint Stiffness: JIA can lead to joint stiffness, making it challenging for children to move their joints, especially after waking up in the morning or after long periods of rest.

4. Fatigue: Many children with JIA feel tired or fatigued, even if they haven't engaged in strenuous activities. This fatigue can affect their daily routines and activities.

5. Fever: Some children with JIA experience intermittent fevers, which may come and go. These fevers are often unrelated to infections and are a result of the body's inflammatory response.

6. Rash: In certain forms of JIA, children may develop a rash on their skin. This rash can vary in appearance but is often red or pink and may be associated with itching.

7. Eye Problems: Chronic uveitis, a type of eye inflammation, can occur in children with JIA. Symptoms may include eye pain, redness, and sensitivity to light.

8. Limited Mobility: Due to joint pain and stiffness, children with JIA may have limited mobility, which can affect their ability to perform daily tasks and participate in physical activities.

9. Growth Issues: In some cases, JIA can affect a child's growth and development, leading to delayed growth or problems with bone development.

10. Emotional and Behavioral Changes: Coping with a chronic condition like JIA can be emotionally challenging for children. They may experience mood swings, anxiety, or depression.

Symptoms for the Various Types of JIA

1. Juvenile enthesitis-related arthritis (ERA)

Some of the symptoms associated with juvenile enthesitis-related arthritis (ERA) include:

- Joint pain, particularly in the knees, hips, ankles, and lower back.

- Joint damage, which can occur over time if not managed.

- Eye inflammation, which can affect vision and eye health.

- Inflammatory bowel disease, which may also be present in some cases.

2. Psoriatic Juvenile Idiopathic Arthritis

Symptoms of this condition can range from mild to severe and may include a combination of the following:

- Swelling in both large and small joints.
- Inflammation at the points where tendons and ligaments attach to bone.

- Swelling of an entire finger or toe.
- Arthritis affecting the lower back or spine.
- Arthritis in the spine.
- Inflammation of the eyes.
- Morning stiffness.
- Back pain or stiffness.
- Pitting or peeling of the nails.
- Redness in the nail beds or cuticles.

3. Systemic Juvenile Idiopathic Arthritis

SJIA is a less common form of JIA, affecting about 10 to 15 percent of all JIA cases. It's characterized by a hyperactive immune system that attacks joints, leading to distinct symptoms:

- Joint Arthritis: SJIA causes joint swelling, along with heat and pain in those affected joints.

- Rashes: Children with SJIA may develop rashes, often accompanied by fever.

- Enlarged Organs: There can be noticeable swelling of lymph nodes or an enlarged liver or spleen.

- Inflammation in Heart or Lungs: SJIA can lead to inflammation in the lining of the heart (pericarditis) or lungs (pleuritis), which can cause discomfort and breathing difficulties.

- Daily Fevers: One of the distinguishing features of SJIA is daily fevers, though they don't usually last for an extended period.

4. Undifferentiated Arthritis

Symptoms of undifferentiated juvenile idiopathic arthritis include:

- Challenges in fully extending the affected leg, arm, or involved joint.
- Alterations in the way a child walks (gait).
- Slow, progressive changes in the jaw's temporomandibular joint, affecting jaw shape, size, and the ability to open the mouth.
- Inflammation of the eyes.
- Occasional high fevers and a rash.
- Limping.

5. Polyarticular Juvenile Idiopathic Arthritis

Children with polyarticular JIA may experience pain, swelling, and stiffness in various joints, and this condition should be addressed with medical attention and care. Additional symptoms include:

- Anemia: This refers to a reduced red blood cell count, which can lead to fatigue and weakness.

- Enlarged Organs: It's possible for the liver, spleen, or lymph nodes to become larger than their normal size.

- Joint Damage: Over time, polyarticular JIA can result in damage to the affected joints, potentially affecting mobility.

- Inflammation in Heart or Lungs: In some cases, this condition can cause inflammation in the lining of the heart or lungs, which may lead to discomfort and breathing difficulties.

6. Oligoarticular juvenile idiopathic arthritis

Additional symptoms that can occur with oligoarticular Juvenile Idiopathic Arthritis (JIA) include:

- Uveitis: This is inflammation inside the eye and, if left untreated, can lead to issues like cataracts, glaucoma, or even blindness.

- Gradual Jaw Changes (Temporomandibular): Over time, there may be changes in the shape and size of the jaw, affecting the ability to fully open the mouth.

- Leg Length Discrepancy: If the knee joint is affected, it could result in one leg being shorter than the other.

- Short Stature: Some children with oligoarticular JIA might be shorter than their peers of the same age who don't have JIA.

It's essential to remember that the symptoms and severity of JIA can vary widely among children. Early diagnosis and appropriate medical care are crucial to managing the condition and improving a child's quality of life. If you suspect your child may have JIA or experience any of these symptoms, it's important to consult a healthcare professional for a proper evaluation and guidance.

Chapter 4

Diagnosis

Diagnosing JIA can be challenging as there isn't a single definitive test for confirmation. The healthcare provider responsible for your child's well-being will carefully review your child's medical history and conduct a thorough physical examination. They will inquire about your child's symptoms and any recent illnesses. JIA diagnosis primarily relies on identifying symptoms of inflammation that have persisted for a duration of six weeks or longer.

Tests may also be done. These include blood tests, imaging tests and other analysis as requested.

Blood Tests

- Antinuclear antibody (ANA) and other antibody tests: These examinations gauge the levels of antibodies in the bloodstream, often associated with rheumatic conditions.

- Complete blood count (CBC): This analysis assesses the counts of red blood cells, white blood cells, and platelets in the blood.

- Complement test: This assessment determines the concentration of complement, a group of blood proteins responsible for eliminating foreign substances. Decreased complement levels are linked to immune-related disorders.

- Erythrocyte sedimentation rate (ESR or sed rate): This test measures how rapidly red blood cells settle at the bottom of a test tube. In the presence of swelling and inflammation, blood proteins cluster together, making them denser than usual. This leads to faster settling of blood cells at the tube's base. The swifter the descent, the more significant the inflammation.

- C-reactive protein (CRP): This protein emerges in response to inflammation in the body. Both ESR and CRP indicate similar levels of inflammation, although one might be elevated when the other isn't. This test may be repeated to evaluate a child's response to medication.

- HLA-B27 testing (a genetic marker): The presence of the HLA-B27 gene is linked to conditions like enthesitis-related arthritis, including ankylosing spondylitis.

- Creatinine: This blood test is conducted to assess kidney function.

- Hematocrit: This measurement determines the quantity of red blood cells in a blood sample. Reduced red blood cell levels (anemia) are frequently observed in individuals with inflammatory arthritis and rheumatic conditions.

- Rheumatoid factor (RF): This examination investigates the presence of RF in the blood, an antibody commonly found in individuals with rheumatoid arthritis and other rheumatic ailments.

- White blood cell count: This measures the number of white blood cells in the blood. Higher levels of white blood cells may mean an infection. Lower levels may be a sign of some rheumatic diseases or a reaction to medicine.

Imaging tests

These examinations can provide information about the extent of bone damage. The tests may comprise:

- X-rays: This procedure employs a minimal amount of radiation to generate images of organs, bones, and other bodily tissues.

- CT scan: This method combines a series of X-ray images with computer technology to create intricate images of bones, muscles, fat, and organs. CT scans offer more detailed views compared to standard X-rays.

- MRI: This diagnostic tool utilizes powerful magnets and computer processing to produce precise images of the body's internal organs and structures.

- Doppler Ultrasound: This specific ultrasound technique is capable of revealing blood flow patterns within the joints, aiding in the identification of areas experiencing inflammation.

- Bone scan: This technique employs a small amount of radiation to accentuate bone features when scanning.

Other tests may include:

- Urine examinations: These tests aim to detect the presence of blood or protein in the urine, which may indicate abnormal kidney function.

- Joint aspiration (arthrocentesis): This involves obtaining a small sample of synovial fluid from a joint to examine for the presence of crystals, bacteria, or viruses.

- Comprehensive eye evaluation conducted by an ophthalmologist.

Consulting Pediatric Rheumatologists

Pediatric Rheumatologists are specialists trained in diagnosing and managing autoimmune and inflammatory conditions in children, including JIA.

Consulting pediatric rheumatologists in cases of JIA (Juvenile Idiopathic Arthritis) is essential due to their specialized expertise in diagnosing and managing this complex condition in children. These experts play a crucial role in the healthcare team, ensuring comprehensive care and improved outcomes for children with JIA.

The necessity of consulting pediatric rheumatologists arises from the unique challenges presented by JIA in children. Unlike adult rheumatoid arthritis, JIA manifests differently in kids and may involve various subtypes, each requiring specific approaches to diagnosis and treatment. Pediatric rheumatologists are trained to recognize these distinctions and provide tailored care.

Their role encompasses several key aspects:

1. Accurate diagnosis: Pediatric rheumatologists are skilled in distinguishing between different forms of arthritis and other conditions that can mimic JIA. Their expertise helps prevent misdiagnosis and ensures that children receive the right treatment promptly.

2. Treatment planning: Once diagnosed, pediatric rheumatologists work closely with the child and their family to develop a customized treatment plan. This may involve a combination of medications, physical therapy, and lifestyle modifications tailored to the child's age, subtype of JIA, and overall health.

3. Medication Management: Pediatric rheumatologists have an in-depth understanding of medications used to manage JIA, including disease-modifying anti-rheumatic drugs (DMARDs) and biologics. They monitor the child's response to these treatments and make necessary adjustments to optimize outcomes while minimizing side effects.

4. Monitoring and Follow-Up: Regular follow-up appointments with pediatric rheumatologists are crucial to track disease progression, address any emerging issues,

and make necessary modifications to the treatment plan. This ongoing care ensures that the child's condition remains well-managed.

5. Pain and Symptom Management: Pediatric rheumatologists also focus on alleviating pain and discomfort associated with JIA, which is vital for a child's overall well-being and quality of life.

6. Education and Support: They educate the child and their family about the condition, its management, and lifestyle factors that can influence JIA. Providing support and guidance is an integral part of their role, helping families navigate the challenges of living with JIA.

Consulting pediatric rheumatologists is imperative in cases of JIA due to their specialized knowledge and experience in managing this condition in children. Their role extends from accurate diagnosis to personalized treatment planning, medication management, monitoring, and ongoing support. This collaborative approach ensures that children with JIA receive comprehensive care tailored to their unique needs, ultimately improving their long-term outcomes and quality of life.

Chapter 5

Treatment Approaches

Although there is no cure for JIA (juvenile idiopathic arthritis), achieving remission, characterized by minimal or no disease activity or symptoms, is a feasible objective. The goal of treatment is to help the child manage discomfort and stiffness while enabling them to maintain as normal a lifestyle as possible. Early and aggressive treatment is crucial for effectively managing the condition.

Furthermore, treatment approaches are individualized based on the child's specific symptoms, age, overall health, and the severity of the condition.

The primary objectives of JIA treatment are as follows:

- Mitigate the long-term health repercussions.
- Prevent damage to joints and organs.
- Maintain joint functionality and mobility.
- Attenuate or halt inflammation.
- Alleviate symptoms, manage pain, and enhance the overall quality of life.
- Attain remission, characterized by minimal or no disease activity or symptoms.

Treatment options may encompass medications, including:

1. Biologic medications: these substances disrupt the body's inflammatory response and come into play when other treatments prove ineffective.

2. Nonsteroidal anti-inflammatory drugs (NSAIDs): these drugs aim to lessen both pain and inflammation.

3. Corticosteroid medications: they are employed to alleviate inflammation and address severe symptoms.

4. Disease-modifying antirheumatic drugs (DMARDs): These medications, including methotrexate, are designed to aid in the reduction of inflammation and the management of JIA (juvenile idiopathic arthritis).

The U.S. Food and Drug Administration (FDA), has granted special approval for over a dozen drugs to treat children with JIA. Nevertheless, your child's physician might also suggest alternative medications.

However, Pediatric rheumatologists have noted that some drugs approved for use in adults appear to be effective in children as well. If your doctor prescribes an adult medication for your child, they might adjust the dosage according to their weight, which is a common practice known as off-label use.

The approved medications for children according to FDA include:

1. Corticosteroids: Prednisone is an approved corticosteroid for children.

2. DMARDs (Disease-Modifying Antirheumatic Drugs): Methotrexate (Trexall, Xatmep) and Sulfasalazine fall into this category and are approved for use in children.

3. Targeted Synthetic DMARD: Tofacitinib is another medication approved for children.

4. NSAIDs: Celecoxib, Ibuprofen (Advil, Motrin), Meloxicam, Naproxen (Aleve), and Tolmetin are non-steroidal anti-inflammatory drugs suitable for children.

5. Biologics: This category includes Abatacept (Orencia), Adalimumab (Humira), Belimumab, Canakinumab, Etanercept (Enbrel, Erelzi, Eticovo), infliximab (Remicade, Inflectra), Golimumab (Simponi), Secukinumab, and Tocilizumab (Actemra).

Some Off-label medications for children include:

- DMARDs: Hydroxychloroquine and Leflunomide are sometimes prescribed to children for conditions not initially intended for.

- Biologics: Anakinra (Kineret), Certolizumab, Infliximab, Rituximab (Rituxan, Truxima, Ruxience) and

Ustekinumab are biologics that may be used for children even if not originally approved for their specific condition.

Additional treatment options and lifestyle adjustments include:

- Regular exercise: Exercise is vital as it enhances both muscle strength and joint flexibility. Swimming stands out as an excellent option because it places minimal strain on your joints.

- Getting enough rest.

- Learning to use large joints instead of small joints to move or carry things.

- Using temperature (heat and cold) therapy: temperature therapy is helpful. Many kids with juvenile idiopathic arthritis experience morning stiffness. Some find relief with cold packs, especially after physical activity. However, most children prefer warmth, like a hot pack, bath, or shower, particularly in the morning.

- Physical therapy, to improve and maintain muscle and joint function.

- Occupational therapy, to improve the ability to do activities of daily living.

- Nutrition: Proper nutrition is essential. Some kids with arthritis might have reduced appetites, while others could gain extra weight due to medications or limited physical

activity. A balanced diet can play a crucial role in
maintaining a healthy body weight.

- Regular eye exams to find early eye changes from
  inflammation.

It is important to note that the pharmaceutical concerns that affect
adults also extend to children, including potential liver problems
caused by methotrexate. Some risks, however, are unique to
children, like the possibility of corticosteroids impeding their
growth. To mitigate these risks, it's crucial to maintain regular
monitoring and open communication with your child's healthcare
provider.

Exciting Future Treatments

This relates to the optimistic outlook in the realm of medical
approaches and therapies currently in development. These hold the
promise of enhancing the well-being of individuals dealing with
conditions such as Juvenile Idiopathic Arthritis (JIA). It's akin to
discovering a beacon of hope at the end of a challenging journey.
These treatments bring the potential for more effective symptom
management, fewer side effects, and an overall improvement in the
quality of life for those affected by JIA. These advancements offer
a peek into a future where patients and their families can look
forward to greater comfort and improved health.

These include:

1. Stem Cell Therapy: Although currently in the early phases of research, stem cell therapy shows promise for regenerating damaged joints in children diagnosed with JIA. Ongoing studies aim to ascertain its safety and efficacy in this context.

2. Precision Medicine: This strategy entails the identification of biomarkers capable of forecasting a child's response to particular JIA treatments. The objective is to tailor treatments for improved results, aligning with each child's unique needs and characteristics.

3. Advanced Biologic Medications: Biologic drugs designed to target precise immune pathways have demonstrated significant potential in effectively managing JIA symptoms. Continual research endeavors are directed towards enhancing current biologics and creating novel ones that offer superior efficacy while minimizing side effects.

4. Immunomodulatory Therapies: Researchers are exploring innovative methods to precisely regulate the immune system's response in JIA. The goal is to diminish inflammation without compromising the overall immune system function.

5. Telemedicine and Remote Monitoring: Progress in telemedicine facilitates remote healthcare access for children with JIA, lessening the necessity for frequent face-to-face appointments. Remote monitoring tools aid in symptom tracking and treatment evaluation.

Chapter 6

Lifestyle and Self-Care

Lifestyle and self-care are closely connected because the choices made within one's lifestyle often dictate the level of self-care required. A healthy lifestyle can reduce the need for self-care in certain areas, but self-care remains vital for maintaining overall well-being and addressing specific needs that may arise in one's life. Both lifestyle and self-care are integral components of a holistic approach to health and well-being, ensuring individuals lead fulfilling and healthy lives.

Lifestyle encompasses the way a person lives their life, influencing their daily routines, habits, and behaviors. It's a comprehensive concept that touches on various aspects of life, including diet, physical activity, sleep patterns, work-life balance, social interactions, and recreational activities.

A healthy lifestyle involves making conscious choices that promote physical, mental, and emotional well-being. This includes eating a balanced diet, engaging in regular exercise, managing stress effectively, getting sufficient sleep, and fostering positive relationships. The choices made in one's lifestyle can have a significant impact on their health and overall quality of life. Adopting a healthy lifestyle is key to preventing various health conditions and improving vitality and longevity.

Self-care on the other hand refers to the deliberate and proactive actions individuals take to care for their physical, emotional, and mental health. It involves recognizing one's own needs and taking steps to meet those needs in order to maintain or restore well-being.

Self-care practices are diverse and tailored to each person's preferences and needs. They can include activities like relaxation techniques, mindfulness, meditation, engaging in hobbies, regular exercise, seeking therapy or counseling when necessary, setting personal boundaries, and allocating time for oneself. Self-care is essential for managing stress, preventing burnout, and cultivating resilience. It allows individuals to recharge, reduce the negative effects of daily stressors, and nurture a healthy sense of self-worth.

Lifestyle in relation to JIA

In the context of Juvenile Idiopathic Arthritis (JIA), lifestyle pertains to the daily choices and routines of children living with this chronic condition. It includes factors such as diet, exercise, sleep patterns, school life, and social activities. For children with JIA, maintaining a healthy lifestyle is particularly important because it can have a direct impact on managing their symptoms and overall well-being.

1. Diet

A balanced diet is essential for children with JIA. Numerous studies indicate that consuming a diet high in fiber can help safeguard against inflammation. It can help manage their weight, which is important because excess weight can strain the joints further. Certain foods, like those rich in anti-inflammatory properties such as fruits and vegetables, can be beneficial in reducing inflammation and alleviating symptoms.

- *Fibres*: Quinoa, sweet potatoes, beans and lentils

- *Protein*: When it comes to sources of protein, it's ideal to prioritize plant-based options like *legumes, beans, peas, lentils, nuts, and seeds*. Additionally, you can consider incorporating protein-rich foods like fatty fish, such as *salmon,* as well as lean cuts of poultry and grass-fed beef into your diet.

- *Foods abundant in omega-3 fatty acids:* Omega-3 fatty acids, which are present in fatty fish like salmon, tuna, and sardines, promote heart health and have anti-inflammatory properties.

- *Fruits and vegetables*: Eating a variety of colorful fruits and vegetables is not only delicious but also beneficial for adults. According to research it prevents chronic diseases. Children taking methotrexate are to incorporate folate-rich dark green leafy vegetables into their diet. Since the medication can lead to deficiencies in this essential nutrient. Some examples of these nutrient-rich foods include: *beets, berries, tomatoes, cherries, broccoli, and kale.*

- *Calcium and vitamin D:* They are essential nutrients for children's health. While both play a crucial role in building strong bones, research indicates that vitamin D also possesses immune-boosting properties. Many children with arthritis often require a combination of calcium and vitamin D supplements," as it is important for children taking corticosteroids and medications like methotrexate, as these drugs may hinder the absorption of calcium - according to Denise Costanzo (a nurse practitioner in the Pediatric Rheumatology Department at the Cleveland Clinic).

- *Herbs and Spices*: According to Jennifer Hyland (a Registered Dietitian Nutritionist (RDN) and a member of the Pediatric Nutrition Support Team at the Cleveland Clinic), herbs and spices can be quite valuable, as many of them have anti-inflammatory properties. Some notable examples include *ginger, turmeric, cinnamon, and rosemary*.

2. Exercise

Physical activity is crucial for children with JIA to maintain joint flexibility and muscle strength. Tailored exercise programs that consider the child's specific condition and limitations are important. These exercises are grouped into two: stretching and strengthening exercises, as they are beneficial for managing pain, reducing stiffness, and preserving mobility.

Stretching exercises:

Stretching is a type of physical activity that entails placing a part of the body in a particular position to enhance muscle flexibility and suppleness. By doing so, it effectively elongates and extends the connected muscle or muscle group.

Here are some gentle stretching exercises suitable for them:

1. *Neck Stretch*:
- Sit or stand up straight.
- Gently tilt your head to one side, bringing your ear closer to your shoulder.
- Hold this position for 10-15 seconds.
- Repeat the stretch on the other side.
- Aim for 2-3 repetitions on each side.

2. *Shoulder Stretch*:
- Sit or stand with a straight back.
- Reach one arm across your chest.
- Use your opposite hand to gently pull your arm closer to your chest.
- Hold for 10-15 seconds.
- Repeat with the other arm.
- Perform 2-3 repetitions for each side.

3. *Arm and Wrist Stretch*:
- Extend one arm straight out in front of you.
- Use your other hand to gently bend your wrist downward.
- Hold for 10-15 seconds.
- Repeat this stretch with the other wrist.
- Do 2-3 repetitions for each wrist.

4. *Chest Opener*:
- Stand with your feet shoulder-width apart.

- Clasp your hands behind your back.
- Slowly pull your arms upward to open your chest.
- Hold for 10-15 seconds.
- Repeat this stretch 2-3 times.

5. *Back Stretch*:
- Sit on the floor with your legs crossed.
- Gently twist your upper body to one side, using your opposite hand to support the twist.
- Hold for 10-15 seconds.
- Repeat on the other side.
- Do 2-3 repetitions on each side.

6. *Hip Flexor Stretch*:
- Kneel on one knee with the other foot in front.
- Carefully shift your weight forward, feeling a stretch in the front of your hip.
- Hold for 10-15 seconds.
- Repeat this stretch with the other leg.
- Perform 2-3 repetitions for each leg.

7. *Quadriceps Stretch*:
- Stand with your feet hip-width apart.
- Bend one knee and bring your heel toward your buttocks.
- Hold your ankle with your hand, gently pulling your heel closer.
- Hold for 10-15 seconds.
- Repeat this stretch with the other leg.
- Do 2-3 repetitions for each leg.

8. *Calf Stretch*:

- Stand facing a wall, with one foot in front of the other.
- Lean forward, keeping your back leg straight and your heel on the ground.
- Hold for 10-15 seconds.
- Repeat with the other leg.
- Complete 2-3 repetitions for each leg.

Emphasize the importance of gentle stretching without forcing any movement. Encourage your child to pay attention to their body and stop any stretch that causes pain. Make stretching a part of their daily routine to maintain joint flexibility and enhance comfort. If you're uncertain, consult with a physical therapist for guidance on suitable stretches tailored to your child's specific condition."

Strengthening exercises:

These are exercises that require your muscles to work harder than their usual level of effort, thereby enhancing your muscles' strength, size, power, and endurance. Strengthening exercises can be categorised into two main types: Isometric and isotonic.

- Isometric exercises

To aid children with Juvenile Idiopathic Arthritis (JIA), it's vital to select gentle exercises that enhance muscle strength and joint stability without overtaxing the affected joints. Below are some suitable isometric exercises:

1. *Static Bridge*: Lie on your back with knees bent and feet flat on the floor. Lift your hips off the ground, creating a

straight line from shoulders to knees. Hold for 5-10 seconds, then release.

2. *Planks*: Support your body on your forearms and toes, keeping your body in a straight line. Hold this position for as long as is comfortable, gradually increasing the time.

3. *Isometric Neck Exercises*: Gently press your hand against your forehead, the side of your head, and the back of your head while resisting the pressure with your neck muscles. Hold each direction for 5-10 seconds.

4. *Isometric Shoulder Press*: Sit or stand with your arms bent at 90 degrees. Push your palms together in front of your chest, engaging your shoulder muscles. Hold for 5-10 seconds.

5. *Knee Press*: Sit on a chair with feet flat on the ground. Press your knees together while engaging your inner thigh muscles. Hold for 5-10 seconds.

6. *Isometric Calf Raises*: Stand with your hands resting on a wall for support. Raise your heels off the ground, engaging your calf muscles. Hold for 5-10 seconds.

7. *Wall Presses*: Stand in front of a wall and gently press your palms against it at chest level. Hold for 5-10 seconds, then release. Repeat several times.

8. *Static Leg Raise*: While lying on your back, raise one leg a few inches off the ground and hold for a count of 5-10 seconds. Switch to the other leg and repeat several times.

9. *Isometric Hand Squeezes*: Use a soft stress ball or sponge and squeeze it with your hand. Hold the squeeze for 5-10 seconds, release, and repeat.

- Isotonic exercises

"It's crucial to pick the right exercises for children dealing with Juvenile Idiopathic Arthritis (JIA). These are exercises that keep their muscles active and their joints moving. The key is to choose activities that are gentle on their joints and match their unique needs. Here are some great isotonic exercises:

1. *Swimming*: Swimming is fantastic for kids with JIA. It's a full-body workout that boosts strength and flexibility without putting too much pressure on their joints.

2. *Cycling*: Whether they're pedaling outdoors or using a stationary bike, cycling is an excellent way to strengthen their leg muscles and improve their overall fitness while being easy on their joints.

3. *Gentle Yoga*: Yoga is great for enhancing flexibility, balance, and muscle strength. Just make sure to pick poses and routines that suit the child's abilities and don't cause any discomfort.

4. *Resistance Bands*: Using resistance bands, kids can do exercises like leg lifts, arm curls, and seated rows to build muscle strength without heavy weights.

5. *Tai Chi*: Tai Chi involves slow, flowing movements that boost balance and flexibility. It's a low-impact choice that works well for kids with JIA.

6. *Pilates*: Pilates focuses on core strength, flexibility, and posture. Modified Pilates exercises can be helpful for kids dealing with JIA.

7. *Balloon Volleyball*: Playing a gentle game of seated or standing balloon volleyball improves hand-eye coordination, upper body strength, and joint mobility.

8. *Low-Impact Aerobics*: Activities like marching in place or following low-impact aerobics videos designed for kids can help improve their cardiovascular fitness.

9. *Seated Leg Lifts*: While sitting down, have the child lift one leg and then the other. This exercise strengthens their leg muscles without putting too much stress on their joints.

10. *Stretching*: Add some gentle stretching exercises to their routine to boost flexibility and keep their joints moving smoothly.

Always make sure a physical therapist or healthcare professional is there to supervise these exercises. They can customize the routine to fit the child's specific needs, keep an eye on their progress, and ensure everything is done safely. The goal is to build strength, flexibility, and overall physical well-being while minimizing any discomfort or risk.

3. School Life

Accommodations may be needed at school to ensure that children with JIA can participate fully. This could include
- additional breaks,
- accessible classrooms, or modified physical education classes.

Self-Care with Relation to JIA

In the context of JIA, self-care focuses on the deliberate actions that children with the condition and their caregivers take to manage symptoms and improve their quality of life.

They include:

1. Medication Management: Children and their caregivers need to adhere to prescribed medication regimens. Understanding the medications, potential side effects, and proper administration is crucial.

2. Pain Management: JIA can cause pain and stiffness in the joints. Self-care practices may include using heat or cold packs to alleviate pain and discomfort. Learning relaxation techniques can also help manage pain.

3. Mental and Emotional Support: Coping with a chronic condition like JIA can be emotionally challenging. Self-care involves seeking emotional support, counseling, and connecting with support groups to address the psychological aspects of the condition.

4. Regular Check-ups: Consistent follow-up with healthcare providers is a form of self-care. It ensures that the child's condition is monitored, and treatment plans can be adjusted if necessary.

5. Safety Precautions: Depending on the severity of JIA, safety measures may be required to prevent injuries. This includes ensuring a safe home environment and using assistive devices when necessary.

6. Sleep: Getting enough quality sleep is vital. Poor sleep can worsen pain and fatigue. Establishing a bedtime routine and addressing any sleep disturbances are important self-care practices.

In summary, for children dealing with Juvenile Idiopathic Arthritis (JIA), lifestyle and self-care go hand in hand. Lifestyle decisions like diet and exercise influence the necessity for self-care in handling symptoms and ensuring overall health. Self-care encompasses daily routines, including medication management, pain relief, emotional support, and regular healthcare, all of which contribute to helping children with JIA lead more comfortable and active lives despite their condition. Both lifestyle choices and self-care are essential aspects of effectively managing JIA and enhancing a child's quality of life.

Chapter 7

Providing Emotional and Psychological Support for Children with JIA

Children who have Juvenile Idiopathic Arthritis (JIA) not only face physical challenges but also emotional and psychological ones. The journey of living with a chronic condition can be overwhelming for both the child and their family.

Emotional and psychological support refers to the help and understanding provided for someone's feelings, emotions, and mental well-being. This support can come from professionals like therapists or counselors, as well as from friends and family. Its primary goal is to assist individuals in coping with various emotional challenges, whether they arise from physical conditions, personal issues, or the normal ups and downs of life.

Children can better handle the emotional challenges tied to their illness when they receive emotional assistance, engage in open conversations, and have access to mental health support. In this part, we'll explore ways to address the emotional effects of JIA, the benefits of counseling and support groups, and methods for nurturing resilience in children.

<h1 style="text-align:center">Dealing with Emotional Impact</h1>

Helping children cope with the emotional toll of Juvenile Idiopathic Arthritis (JIA) demands a caring and empathetic approach. Here are some approaches to assist children cope with the emotional challenges of JIA:

Open Communication

- Encourage your child to share their feelings and worries. Make it clear that discussing emotions is perfectly okay.
- Be a good listener, offering a safe and non-judgmental space for them to express themselves.
- Explain their condition and treatment using language suitable for their age, helping them grasp what lies ahead.

Normalize Emotions

- Assure your child that it's absolutely normal to experience a range of emotions, like frustration, sadness, anger, or fear.
- Share stories of other children with JIA who have successfully managed their condition and lead fulfilling lives.

Supportive Environment

- Cultivate a loving and accepting home environment where children feel secure and cherished, no matter their health condition.

- Involve the entire family in understanding and supporting the child with JIA.

Education

- Educate your child about JIA and its management. Knowledge can alleviate anxiety and uncertainty.
- Utilize educational materials, books, or online resources specifically designed for children with JIA.

Encourage Independence

- Empower your child to actively participate in managing their condition as they grow. This instills a sense of control.
- Celebrate their achievements, however small, to boost their self-esteem.

Professional Help

- Consider involving a child psychologist or therapist specializing in chronic illnesses. They can offer coping strategies and emotional support.
- If your child's emotional distress is significant, therapy may be beneficial.

Peer Support

- Motivate your child to connect with peers who share similar conditions. Support groups or online communities can be incredibly valuable.

- These connections help children understand they're not alone and foster a sense of belonging.

Stress Reduction

- Teach your child relaxation techniques like deep breathing, meditation, or mindfulness to manage stress and anxiety.

Positive Outlook

- Foster a positive attitude by focusing on your child's strengths and capabilities, not just their limitations.
- Emphasize that JIA doesn't define who they are as a person.

Regular Check-Ins

- Periodically check in with your child about their emotional well-being. Ask how they're feeling and if they need additional support.

Every child's reaction to JIA is unique, so it's crucial to be patient, adaptable, and compassionate. By creating a supportive and empathetic atmosphere, you can guide your child through the emotional difficulties of living with JIA and help them develop resilience for the future.

Counseling and Support Groups

Counseling and support groups play a crucial role in the lives of children and families dealing with Juvenile Idiopathic Arthritis

(JIA). These services provide a lifeline for children with JIA, offering a safe and understanding environment where they can openly discuss their emotions and fears related to their chronic condition.

While support groups create connections among families on similar journeys, fostering a sense of community and shared experiences, professional counseling offers specialized guidance to help children develop effective coping strategies and emotional resilience.

The combination of counseling and support groups empowers children with JIA and their families, enabling them to confront both the physical and emotional challenges of the condition with strength and confidence. Ultimately, these services contribute to enhancing the overall quality of life for those affected by JIA.

Professional counselling

Seeking professional counseling at times can be helpful. Therapists or counselors can provide coping strategies, stress management techniques, and a supportive environment for children to talk about their emotions.

This can be done through various avenues:

1. Pediatric Rheumatologist or Healthcare Provider: Start by discussing your child's emotional needs with their pediatric rheumatologist or primary healthcare provider. They can provide referrals to mental health professionals who

specialize in working with children dealing with chronic illnesses.

2. Children's Hospitals and Medical Centers: Many large children's hospitals and medical centers employ pediatric psychologists or child life specialists experienced in counseling children with chronic conditions like JIA. Inquire about these services at your child's healthcare facility.

3. Local Mental Health Clinics: Explore local mental health clinics, as they may have child psychologists or therapists who can provide counseling for children with chronic illnesses. Contact these clinics to inquire about their services and expertise in dealing with JIA.

4. Schools: School counselors can be a valuable resource, offering support to children with chronic conditions. They may also have recommendations for additional counseling services if needed.

5. Online Resources: Telehealth services have become more accessible. Some child psychologists and therapists offer online counseling sessions, providing convenience for families without easy access to in-person services.

6. Pediatric Rheumatology Centers: Specialized pediatric rheumatology centers or research institutions may include counselors or psychologists as part of their multidisciplinary teams.

7. Support Organizations: Reach out to organizations such as the Arthritis Foundation, JIA Foundation, or local arthritis support groups. They can offer information on available counseling services and resources in your area.

8. Insurance Provider: Check with your health insurance provider to understand your coverage for mental health services. They may maintain a list of covered providers that you can contact.

When seeking professional counseling for your child with JIA, prioritize finding a therapist or psychologist with experience in pediatric chronic illnesses. They should be capable of working with your child to address their specific emotional needs related to JIA and help them develop effective coping strategies. As a parent, advocate for your child's well-being, and don't hesitate to explore different options until you find the right fit for your family's needs.

Support groups

Support groups specifically designed for children with JIA can be incredibly valuable. They offer a sense of belonging and understanding that can be difficult to find elsewhere. Encourage your child to participate in these groups, whether in person or online.

Here are some organizations and support groups focused on JIA:

1. Arthritis Foundation
- The Arthritis Foundation provides a range of resources and programs for children with JIA and their families. They may have local p that organize support groups and events.
- Website: https://www.arthritis.org/diseases/juvenile-arthritis

2. Kids Get Arthritis Too
- This program, part of the Arthritis Foundation, is specifically designed for children and teenagers with arthritis. They offer resources, events, and online communities.
- Website: https://www.kidsgetarthritistoo.org/

3. CARRA (Children's Arthritis and Rheumatology Research Alliance)
- CARRA is a collaborative group of pediatric rheumatologists, researchers, and families working to enhance the care of children with rheumatic conditions, including JIA.
- Website: https://www.carragroup.org/

4. JIA-at-NRAS (National Rheumatoid Arthritis Society)
- Although based in the UK, JIA-at-NRAS provides information and support to children and young people dealing with Juvenile Idiopathic Arthritis.

- Website:
  https://www.jia.org.uk/

5. JIA Foundation
- The JIA Foundation is dedicated to improving the lives of children with JIA through research, awareness, and support. They offer information and resources for families.
- Website:
  https://jiafoundation.org/

6. Cure JM Foundation
- While primarily focused on Juvenile Myositis, an autoimmune disease, the Cure JM Foundation provides resources and support for families dealing with various pediatric rheumatic conditions, including JIA.
- Website:
  https://curejm.org/

7. ACR (American College of Rheumatology) Rheumatology Research Foundation
- ACR's Rheumatology Research Foundation supports research and advocacy for various rheumatic diseases, including those affecting children. They offer educational materials and resources.
- Website:
  https://www.rheumresearch.org/

8. Local Hospitals and Clinics
- Many hospitals and pediatric rheumatology clinics organize support groups or connect families facing JIA.

Check with your local healthcare providers for resources in your area.

9. Online Communities
- Online forums and social media groups can also serve as valuable sources of support. Websites like Inspire and PatientsLikeMe host communities dedicated to JIA.

Please keep in mind that the availability of support groups may vary depending on your location. To learn more about local support groups, events, and resources, consider reaching out to these organizations or visiting their websites. Additionally, consulting your child's healthcare provider can provide guidance on JIA-specific support available in your region.

Fostering Resilience in Children with JIA

Resilience means being able to recover from difficulties and setbacks, and it's an important quality for children with JIA as they navigate the ups and downs of life. Children must develop resilience in order to effectively handle life's challenges and mature into emotionally and mentally strong adults. Resilient children can adapt to tough situations, manage them, and bounce back.

These strategies can assist young individuals in cultivating resilience:

- Cultivate a Positive Mindset: Teach your child to focus on their strengths and achievements rather than limitations. Foster optimism and a "can-do" attitude.

- Promote Self-Care: Highlight the importance of self-care, including adequate rest, nutrition, and exercise. These habits contribute to both physical and emotional well-being.

- Building Problem-Solving Skills: Help your child develop problem-solving abilities. Teach them how to break challenges into manageable steps and find solutions. This will enhance adaptability and self-confidence.

- Creating a Supportive Environment: Establish a home environment where your child feels loved, accepted, and encouraged to pursue their goals.

- Support independence: This involves providing children with chances to make decisions suitable for their age. This helps boost their self-esteem and gives them a sense of control.

- Nurture a growth mindset: to do this you have to consistently highlight that abilities and intelligence can grow through effort and learning, and encouraging them to embrace this perspective.

- Encourage Expression through Art and Play: Supporting children to express their emotions through activities like art, music, and play can create a safe and nurturing space for them.

- Seeking Professional Guidance: If necessary, consult with a child psychologist or therapist who specializes in chronic illnesses to work on resilience-building strategies.

Remember, providing emotional and psychological support is an ongoing process. Be patient with your child and yourself. Together, you can navigate the emotional impact of JIA and nurture resilience for a brighter future.

Chapter 8

Family and Caregiver Support for Children with Rheumatoid Arthritis (RA)

Support from family and caregivers for children dealing with Rheumatoid Arthritis (RA) encompasses various aspects. It includes emotional, practical, and educational assistance offered by family members and caregivers to the child living with RA.

This support involves nurturing a compassionate and understanding atmosphere at home, educating family members about the condition and how to manage it, providing emotional reassurance to the child, and adapting daily routines to accommodate the child's requirements.

Such support plays a vital role in aiding the child in dealing with the challenges presented by RA and promoting their overall health and happiness. In this section, we'll delve into effective approaches for parents, siblings, and caregivers to offer optimal support and comprehension.

Parenting a Child with Rheumatoid Arthritis

Parenting a child with Rheumatoid Arthritis (RA) can be a challenging journey that affects not only the child with the condition but the entire family. Parenting a child with RA involves a delicate balance of providing physical care and emotional support.

Parents should:

- Educate themselves about RA and its management.

- Foster open communication with their child, encouraging them to express their feelings and concerns.

- Create a supportive and inclusive family environment where the child feels loved and accepted.

- Understand that your child may experience pain, frustration, and limitations. Be patient and empathetic in your interactions.

- Be an advocate for your child within the healthcare system. Ensure they receive appropriate care and accommodations.

- Collaborate closely with healthcare providers to ensure optimal treatment.

Sibling Support and Understanding

Siblings of children with RA may have unique emotional experiences.

It's essential to:

- Educate siblings about RA to demystify the condition.

- Encourage open dialogue, allowing siblings to ask questions and share their feelings.

- Keep an eye out for any signs of bullying or discrimination. Encourage your child to communicate openly with you about what happens outside the home, and provide guidance on how to handle these situations.

- Allocate one-on-one time with each sibling to maintain a sense of normalcy.

- Acknowledge the emotional challenges siblings may face and offer support.

- Some organizations offer support groups specifically for siblings of children with chronic illnesses. Consider exploring these resources.

Balancing Caregiving with Other Responsibilities

Balancing caregiving responsibilities for a child with RA with other life commitments can be demanding. But the following will help in the execution of this task.

Caregivers should:

- Seek support from family members, friends, or support groups.

- Create a flexible schedule that accommodates medical appointments and treatments.

- Prioritize self-care to prevent caregiver burnout.

- Communicate openly with employers or schools about the child's condition to ensure understanding and flexibility.

- If caregiving becomes overwhelming, consider seeking professional guidance or counseling to manage stress and emotional challenges.

In providing support as parents, siblings, or caregivers, it's crucial to remember that RA affects the entire family. By fostering understanding, open communication, and a nurturing environment, families can navigate the challenges of RA together, promoting the well-being of their child and each other.

Chapter 10

FAQs on JIA

Here are 35 frequently asked questions (FAQs) about Juvenile Idiopathic Arthritis (JIA):

1. What is Juvenile Idiopathic Arthritis (JIA)?

JIA is a chronic autoimmune disease that causes joint inflammation in children and adolescents under the age of 16.

2. How common is JIA?

JIA is relatively rare but is the most common form of arthritis in children, affecting about 1 in 1,000 children.

3. What causes JIA?

The exact cause is unknown, but it's believed to involve a combination of genetic and environmental factors triggering an autoimmune response.

4. What are the common symptoms of JIA?

Common symptoms include joint pain, swelling, stiffness, fatigue, and reduced mobility. Some forms of JIA may also cause eye inflammation, skin rashes, or fever.

5. *Is JIA the same as adult rheumatoid arthritis (RA)?*

No, JIA is a distinct condition. While they share similarities, they have differences in symptoms, prognosis, and treatment.

6. *How is JIA diagnosed?*

Diagnosis involves a combination of medical history, physical examination, blood tests, and imaging. A pediatric rheumatologist typically confirms the diagnosis.

7. *Can JIA go into remission?*

Yes, with early and effective treatment, JIA can go into remission. However, it can also flare up again.

8. *What are the treatment options for JIA?*

Treatment may include medications to reduce inflammation, physical and occupational therapy, lifestyle modifications, and, in some cases, surgery.

9. *Can children with JIA lead normal lives?*

Yes, many children with JIA can lead normal lives with appropriate treatment and support.

10. *Are there different types of JIA?*

Yes, there are several subtypes of JIA, each with distinct characteristics and treatment approaches.

11. Is JIA a lifelong condition?

It varies from person to person. Some children may outgrow JIA, while others may continue to experience symptoms into adulthood.

12. How can I support a child with JIA?

Offer emotional support, educate yourself about the condition, and collaborate closely with healthcare providers.

13. Can diet or lifestyle changes help manage JIA symptoms?

While a balanced diet and exercise are important for overall health, specific dietary changes should be discussed with a healthcare provider.

14. Are there support groups for families dealing with JIA?

Yes, there are support groups and organizations dedicated to JIA that offer resources, information, and connections with other families.

15. Can children with JIA participate in sports and physical activities?

Many children with JIA can engage in sports and physical activities with modifications and guidance from healthcare professionals.

16. What's the long-term outlook for children with JIA?

With early diagnosis and appropriate treatment, many children with JIA can lead fulfilling lives with minimal joint damage.

17. Can JIA affect a child's schooling?

Yes, JIA may affect school attendance and participation. Schools should be informed about the condition to provide necessary accommodations.

18. Are there medications specifically for JIA?

Yes, there are medications designed to manage JIA symptoms and reduce inflammation, including nonsteroidal anti-inflammatory drugs (NSAIDs) and biologics.

19. Can JIA cause disability?

While JIA can cause joint damage, early intervention and proper treatment can often prevent significant disability.

20. Are there any alternative or complementary therapies for JIA?

Some families explore complementary therapies like acupuncture or dietary supplements, but these should be discussed with a healthcare provider.

21. What is the role of physical therapy in JIA management?

Physical therapy helps improve joint mobility, muscle strength, and overall function in children with JIA.

22. How often should a child with JIA see their rheumatologist?

The frequency of visits depends on the child's specific condition and treatment plan, but regular follow-up is essential.

23. Can stress worsen JIA symptoms?

Stress can potentially trigger symptom flares, so managing stress is important for children with JIA.

24. Are there clinical trials for JIA treatments?

Yes, there are ongoing clinical trials researching new treatments and therapies for JIA. A healthcare provider can provide information on available trials.

25. Where can I find reliable information about JIA?

Reputable sources include pediatric rheumatology clinics, healthcare providers, organizations like the Arthritis Foundation, and medical literature.

26. Are there any lifestyle tips for managing JIA symptoms?

Maintaining a balanced lifestyle with regular exercise, a healthy diet, and adequate sleep can help manage JIA symptoms.

27. Can JIA affect a child's growth and development?

In some cases, JIA can impact growth and development. Regular monitoring by healthcare providers can address these concerns.

28. How can I explain JIA to my child's classmates and friends?

Educate classmates and friends about JIA to foster understanding. Encourage open conversations and provide age-appropriate information.

29. Can children with JIA travel or participate in outdoor activities?

Yes, with proper planning and accommodations, children with JIA can enjoy travel and outdoor activities like camping and hiking.

30. Is there a cure for JIA?

While there is no cure, effective management and treatment can help control symptoms and improve the child's quality of life.

31. Can children with JIA attend regular schools?

Many children with JIA attend regular schools with support and accommodations. It's essential to work with the school to ensure the child's needs are met.

32. Are there JIA-specific organizations or camps for children?

Yes, there are organizations that offer camps and events tailored to children with JIA, providing opportunities for socialization and support.

33. Can JIA affect a child's mental health?

Coping with a chronic condition can impact a child's mental health. Regular communication with healthcare providers can address emotional well-being.

34. How can I help my child transition to adult care as they grow older?

Transition planning involves working with healthcare providers to ensure a seamless move from pediatric to adult rheumatology care.

35. Are there assistive devices that can help children with JIA?

Yes, assistive devices like splints, braces, or mobility aids may be recommended to support joint function and mobility.

These FAQs provide a comprehensive overview of Juvenile Idiopathic Arthritis, but it's essential to consult with healthcare professionals for personalized guidance and information related to your child's specific situation.

Conclusion

In the voyage through childhood Rheumatoid Arthritis (RA), a powerful force emerges – hope. As we wrap up our exploration of RA in children, we stress the significance of empowerment and the bright future it promises. Empowering these young individuals goes beyond managing their medical condition; it's about nurturing their dreams, supporting their ambitions, and fostering their resilience.

With advancements in research, medical treatments, and holistic support, we're paving the way for children with RA to thrive. It's a future where they can pursue their passions, achieve their goals, and confront life's challenges with unwavering determination. RA may be a chapter in their story, but it doesn't define them.

As caregivers, healthcare providers, and advocates, it's our shared duty to equip these children with the tools for success. Together, we're crafting a future where hope conquers adversity, possibilities are limitless, and every child with RA can reach their full potential.

Let's continue working hand in hand, nurturing a future filled with hope, resilience, and boundless opportunities for these incredible children living with Rheumatoid Arthritis. Their journey showcases the indomitable human spirit, and their future shines with endless hope.

References

https://carle.org/conditions/rheumatoid-arthritis-juvenile

https://medlineplus.gov/genetics/condition/juvenile-idiopathic-arthritis/

https://rheumatology.org/patients/juvenile-arthritis

https://www.aboutkidshealth.ca/https://www.arthritis.org/diseases/juvenile-arthritis

https://www.arthritis.org/diseases/juvenile-arthritis

https://www.arthritis.org/diseases/juvenile-idiopathic-arthritis

https://www.arthritis.org/diseases/systemic-juvenile-idiopathic-arthritis

https://www.carragroup.org/

https://www.cdc.gov/arthritis/types/childhood.htm

https://www.everydayhealth.com/rheumatoid-arthritis/juvenile-idiopathic-arthritis-signs-and-symptoms/

https://www.hopkinsmedicine.org/health/conditions-and-diseases/arthritis/juvenile-idiopathic-arthritis

https://www.jrd.or.kr/journal/view.html?doi=10.4078/jrd.2018.25.4.221

https://www.kidsgetarthritistoo.org/

https://www.mayoclinic.org/diseases-conditions/juvenile-idiopathic-arthritis/diagnosis-treatment/drc-20374088

https://www.ncbi.nlm.nih.gov/pmc/articles/PMC8638433/

https://www.nhs.uk/live-well/exercise/strength-and-flexibility-exercises/how-to-improve-strength-flexibility/

https://www.niams.nih.gov/health-topics/juvenile-arthritis

https://www.niams.nih.gov/health-topics/juvenile-arthritis

https://www.physio-pedia.com/Stretching#cite_note-1

https://www.uptodate.com/contents/undifferentiated-early-inflammatory-arthritis-in-adults/print#

https://www.verywellhealth.com/what-is-undifferentiated-arthritis-189641

https://www.yalemedicine.org/conditions/juvenile-idiopathic-arthritis

https://www.yummymummyclub.ca/blogs/dr-kim-foster-wicked-health/20150306/could-your-child-have-arthritis

Schiff, M. H. (2010). Preventing the progression from undifferentiated arthritis to rheumatoid arthritis: the clinical and economic implications. *Am J Manag Care.* Nov; 16(9 Suppl):S243-8. PMID: 21517637.

www.ingramcontent.com/pod-product-compliance
Lightning Source LLC
Chambersburg PA
CBHW060755260726
48660CB00002B/627